From Stress to Serenity:

Spiritual Techniques for Emotional Balance

Published by: Jake A. Waldron

I0838018

Jake A Waldron

COPY RIGHT © 2024 by Jake A. Waldron

TABLE OF CONTENTS

INTRODUCTION

Stress has become an all-too-common companion for many in today's fast-paced society. Recent research indicates that around 80% of Americans consistently feel stress, which negatively affects their mental and physical health. We may feel overburdened and exhausted by the constant demands of our families, jobs, and society. This book extends an invitation to go on a transforming voyage from tension to tranquility, delving into the significant influence of emotional equilibrium and the spiritual practices that can direct you on this route.

The Value of Maintaining Emotional Balance

Maintaining emotional equilibrium is not only a luxury; it's essential to living a happy life. It enables us to sustain wholesome relationships, develop a feeling of purpose, and face obstacles head-on. When we are in balance emotionally, we are more capable of handling hardship, making wise choices, and finding happiness in the little things in life. But striking this balance is frequently easier said than done, particularly in a world where there are many diversions and life moves at a constant tempo.

The Road Ahead

This book provides a thorough overview of spiritual practices that can assist you in achieving emotional equilibrium. Through a variety of techniques, including yoga, mindfulness, meditation, and prayer, you'll learn effective strategies to reduce stress and improve your emotional health. Every chapter explores a particular method in detail, offering you doable instructions, insightful analysis, and true anecdotes that highlight the practices' transforming potential.

We will examine the nature of stress in Chapter 1, looking at its several forms and the significant impacts it can have on our mental, emotional, and physical well-being. The first step to dealing with stress, is recognizing it.

In Chapter 2, the relationship between spirituality and emotional health will be discussed, along with how spiritual activities help build resilience. We will examine empirical research that shows how spirituality can help people feel less stressed and more at peace with themselves.

We will then start delving deeply into each practice individually. You will be guided through various spiritual practices in each chapter, which will include insights, useful exercises, and integration tips for your everyday life. You will discover approachable and enlightening ways to develop serenity, whether it's through mindfulness (Chapter 5) or the curative effects of prayer (Chapter 4).

Individual Narratives of Metamorphosis

You will come across first-hand accounts on this journey from people who have successfully made the transition from stress to calm. These true stories will motivate you and teach you important lessons about resiliency and recovery. Think about how their stories might relate to your own as you read about their experiences.

Taking Part in the Community

Relationships with other people frequently improve one's emotional health. Building a strong spiritual community is crucial, and Chapter 11 will show how interacting with like-minded people may create a feeling of community and purpose. This sense of belonging can be a really useful tool for you on your trip.

A Call to Action

I urge you to approach this journey with an open mind and heart as you set out on it. Consider your personal encounters with emotional equilibrium and stress. What challenges do you face? Which of the practices you have tried seem to be most effective for you? You will be encouraged to think and participate in every chapter, which will help you gain a better knowledge of your personal path to tranquility.

You will find inspiration, useful advice, and a plethora of knowledge in the pages that follow. I hope that this book will be a reliable guide for you as you investigate spiritual methods that can change the way you relate to stress and lead you from chaos to peace.

Chapter 1

Understanding Stress and Its Impact on Emotional Health

Stress is a common occurrence that impacts people from all different backgrounds. It can have a big impact on our mental, emotional, and physical health and can take many different forms. This chapter will define stress, look at its various forms, analyze its impacts, and talk about how persistent stress might thwart our efforts to achieve emotional equilibrium.

What Stress Is

In essence, stress is the body's reaction to stressors—perceived dangers or difficulties. These might be internal, like negative thoughts or self-imposed pressures, or external, such relationship problems or work deadlines. Stress sets off a complicated physiological reaction that is commonly known as the "fight-or-flight" response, during which the body releases large amounts of cortisol and adrenaline. While in short spurts this response

From Stress to Serenity: Spiritual Techniques for Emotional Balance
might be useful, enabling us to respond quickly to danger, persistent stress
can result in serious health problems.

Stress Types

It is essential to comprehend the many forms of stress in order to
effectively manage:

1. **Acute Stress**: This type is the most prevalent and usually results
   from recent experiences. While it can be thrilling and inspiring, if
   unchecked, it can build up and cause anxiety.

2. **Chronic Stress**: Unlike acute stress, chronic stress is more
   persistent. It may be the result of persistent life difficulties
   including unresolved interpersonal conflicts or money troubles.
   Prolonged stress can have catastrophic consequences for one's
   physical and mental well-being.

3. **Eustress**: This type of stress may be energizing and motivating.
   As an illustration, consider getting ready for a significant occasion,
   beginning a new work, or taking a long-awaited vacation.

4. Distress: This is the harmful kind of stress that can become
   overwhelming and impair our ability to function. It frequently
   happens as a result of circumstances that seem dangerous or
   uncontrollable.

Stress's Physical, Mental, and Emotional Effects

Numerous mechanisms exist for stress to appear in several areas of health:

1. **Physical Effects**: Prolonged stress can cause a host of health problems, such as heart disease, digestive disorders, headaches, and weakened immune systems. The body may become strained due to the continuous release of stress hormones, which can result in physical problems such as weariness.

2. **Effects on the Mind**: Excessive stress can hinder mental abilities including focus, memory, and decision-making. Additionally, it may raise the chance of mental health conditions like depression and anxiety.

3. **Effects on Emotions**: Emotional instability is frequently brought on by stress. It is possible for people to feel agitated, frustrated, or depressed. Persistent stress can cause a person to lose motivation and feel powerless.

Persistent Stress's Effects on Everything Health and Welfare

The long-term consequences of persistent stress are significant. Prolonged activation of the stress response in the body can upset homeostasis over time and cause a number of problems. Persistent stress can worsen pre-existing diseases, lead to burnout, and damage relationships. Additionally, stress can lead to unhealthy coping strategies like overeating, substance abuse, or social disengagement, which can exacerbate preexisting mental and physical health conditions.

Take into consideration the narrative of Sarah, a young professional who experienced ongoing stress, to demonstrate these ideas. She started having frequent migraines, exhaustion, and anxiety due to the pressures of her personal and professional lives being too much for her. She tried working more hours to help herself, but she felt stuck in a stressful cycle that made her symptoms worse. Her journey towards emotional equilibrium and overall wellbeing only started when she started looking for assistance and investigating spiritual traditions.

Indices of Stress

Effective stress management requires an understanding of the symptoms of stress. Typical signs and symptoms include:

- **Emotional Symptoms**: Increased irritation, anxiety, mood swings, and feelings of overload.

- **Physical:** headaches, soreness in the muscles, exhaustion, irregular sleep patterns, and stomach problems.

- **Behavioral Symptoms**: Changes in appetite, retreat from social activities, and difficulties concentrating.

By spotting these signals early, you can take proactive efforts to treat stress before it escalates.

In summary

Understanding stress is the first step toward handling it properly. You give yourself the power to take action by identifying the different forms of stress, realizing its extensive impacts, and identifying personal symptoms. We'll look at spiritual strategies in the upcoming chapters that can help you change the way you relate to stress and start along the path to emotional equilibrium and tranquility.

Consider journaling to record your feelings, triggers, and reactions as you think back on your personal experiences with stress. As you navigate the upcoming problems, this practice might offer insightful information. Remember that awareness and comprehension are the first steps on the way to serenity.

.

Chapter 2

The Connection Between Spirituality and Emotional Well-being

A strong ally in our search for emotional equilibrium is frequently spirituality. Although everyone's definition of spirituality is unique and can be quite personal, it alludes to a feeling of being connected to something bigger than ourselves. This chapter delves into the complex interrelationships that exist between spirituality and emotional health, the ways in which spiritual practices can strengthen resilience, and the empirical evidence supporting these relationships.

Spirituality Definition

A broad definition of spirituality encompasses human development, religious beliefs, and the pursuit of meaning and purpose. It frequently entails reflection and the search for a more profound comprehension of oneself and one's role in the cosmos. There are many other ways that spirituality can appear, such as through acts of compassion, organized religion, nature, meditation, and creative expression. In contrast to religion, which frequently adheres to a certain theory or body of beliefs, spirituality is more flexible and personalized. It provides direction and a feeling of purpose in an increasingly chaotic world, allowing for individual interpretation and the ability to change over time.

The Significance of Spirituality in Mental Health:

A rising body of research backs up the notion that spirituality might be extremely important for mental health. The following are some important domains in which spirituality is beneficial:

1. **Coping Mechanism**: Spirituality can give people a foundation for comprehending and resolving the difficulties in life. People who rely on spiritual ideas frequently find solace in the notion that they are a part of a greater scheme or purpose, which helps lessen depressing feelings of loneliness.

2. **Emotional Resilience:** Research indicates that engaging in spiritual activities like meditation or prayer might improve emotional resilience. They help people manage pressures more skillfully by promoting a positive outlook, lowering anxiety, and cultivating a sense of serenity.

3. **Social Support:** Becoming involved in spiritual communities, whether via nature clubs, religious organizations, or meditation groups, can provide one a sense of support and belonging. This social interaction is essential for mental health because it fosters emotional stability and lessens feelings of loneliness.

4. **Mindfulness and Presence:** Being able to stay fully present and involved in the moment is emphasized in many spiritual practices. It has been demonstrated that practicing mindfulness lowers stress and improves emotional control, which increases feelings of calm.

Research on Spirituality and Stress Reduction in Science

Numerous research have looked into the connection between mental health and spirituality. Here are some noteworthy discoveries:

- According to a research in the **Journal of Health Psychology**, people who regularly practice spirituality report feeling less stressed and more satisfied with their lives. The study found that coping mechanisms that spirituality offers help people become resilient in the face of hardship.

- The **American Psychological Association's** research suggests that spirituality can result in improved health outcomes. Individuals who self-identified as spiritual or religious showed reduced anxiety and depression levels in contrast to those who did not.

- **A University of California study** discovered that participants' cortisol levels—a stress marker—were considerably lowered by mindfulness meditation, a popular spiritual practice. Regular mindfulness practitioners reported feeling more emotionally stable and well-being.

Spiritual Exercises' Beneficial Effects on Emotional Resilience

The ability to adjust to pressure, hardship, trauma, and tragedy is known as emotional resilience. It entails rising above trying circumstances and retaining optimism in the face of adversity. Spiritual activities can greatly increase this resilience by giving people the tools and frameworks they need to deal with the challenges of life. Here is a closer examination of the ways in which particular spiritual activities support emotional fortitude.

1. Meditation

A fundamental spiritual practice that fosters emotional resilience in a number of ways is meditation.

➢ Meditation fosters mindfulness and awareness by keeping one's attention on the here and now. This awareness lowers reactivity and improves emotional regulation by enabling people to watch their ideas and feelings without passing judgment. People who frequently meditate are more likely to react rationally rather than impulsively while under stress.

➢ **Reduced Stress**: Studies show that meditation can reduce cortisol levels, which are a sign of stress. Not only does this decrease in stress enhance mental health overall, but it also better prepares people to deal with stress in the future.

➢ **Enhanced Self-Compassion**: A key component of emotional resilience, meditation cultivates self-compassion. People who practice self-kindness are better able to handle mistakes because they see them as a natural part of life rather than as personal failings.

2. Prayer

A very private spiritual practice that has a significant impact on emotional resilience is prayer:

➢ **Community and Connection**: Prayer helps many people feel a part of a larger group or a higher power. This connection can promote a sense of belonging and lessen feelings of loneliness, both of which are important during trying times.

➢ **Emotional Release**: You can communicate your hopes, worries, and thanks through prayer. Emotional processing is facilitated by the act of vocalizing sentiments, which also serves as a therapeutic release that improves emotional resilience and clarity.

> ➤ **A Shift in Perspective**: Praying often inspires people to consider their problems from a different angle. This change in perspective can help people feel hopeful and trust that things will get better, which is essential for resilience.

3. Acts of Gratitude

One effective spiritual practice that can change how people react to tragedy is cultivating gratitude:

> ➤ Positive Reframing: Thinking back on what you have to be thankful for on a regular basis promotes optimism and helps people reframe their circumstances. This constructive rephrasing can help reduce tension and anxiety, promoting a more stable emotional state.

> ➤ Building Resilience via Recognition: Practicing gratitude helps people stay aware of their blessings and support system, especially in the face of adversity. This recognition can strengthen resilience by fostering optimism and fortitude.

> ➤ Community and Connection: Being grateful frequently entails appreciating the efforts of others, which fortifies bonds and creates a network of support. Resilience depends on having strong social ties since these relationships offer emotional support through trying times.

4. The Connection to Nature

Being in nature is a spiritual activity that strengthens emotional fortitude:

> ➤ The restorative effects of being outside have been demonstrated to lower stress and elevate happiness. Natural environments have a calming influence that helps people rediscover who they are and how big their problems really are.

- ➤ **Mindfulness in Nature:** Engaging in outdoor activities such as hiking, gardening, or park strolling fosters mindfulness, enhancing presence and awareness. This sense of groundedness that comes from being connected to nature might help people feel at ease during turbulent times.
- ➤ **Sense of Belonging:** Being in nature frequently makes one feel as though they are a part of their surroundings. Emotional resilience can be strengthened by this feeling of support and strength from something greater than oneself.

5. Expression of Creativity

Engaging in creative endeavors can function as potent spiritual exercises that enhance emotional fortitude:

- ➤ **Self-Discovery and Processing:** Creating art, music, writing, or dancing enables people to communicate feelings that they might find hard to put into words. Making meaning of experiences and emotions is facilitated by this creative outlet, which acts as a kind of emotional processing.
- ➤ **Empowerment:** The process of producing gives people a sense of agency and control. Knowing that one is capable of creating and expressing oneself can be a source of strength in the face of difficulty.
- ➤ **Community and Connection:** Working together or sharing with others is a common aspect of creative pursuits. Social support is a key element of emotional resilience, and this link can strengthen it.

6. Customs and Traditions

Creating spiritual routines can help bring emotional resilience the structure and consistency it needs:

- ➤ **Sense of Stability:** Consistent spiritual practices, such weekly meetings, morning meditations, or seasonal celebrations, foster a sense of stability. In turbulent times, this regularity can provide a sense of stability.

> ➤ **Reflective practices:** Rituals frequently promote introspection, enabling people to evaluate their feelings and encounters. By encouraging introspection, people become more self-aware and are able to recognize patterns in their reactions to stress.
> ➤ **Community ties:** Engaging in collective customs fortifies interpersonal relationships and establishes a network of assistance. Being able to rely on a community promotes resilience since shared experiences and group support can act as a stress reliever.

Enhancing emotional resilience can be greatly facilitated by engaging in spiritual practices. Through the cultivation of mindfulness, connection, gratitude, and self-expression, these practices empower people to face life's obstacles with more ease and self-assurance. Examine how the several spiritual practices in this book can improve your emotional forbearance and lead to a more tranquil, well-balanced life as you study them.

We will go into more detail about meditation as a route to inner peace in the upcoming chapter, providing helpful advice to get you started and keep up a rewarding practice. Your spiritual practices can be important friends in your path to emotional well-being, so think about your personal beliefs and which ones speak to you the most.

Cultural Views on Spirituality and Mental Wellness

A fundamental part of human existence, spirituality is greatly influenced by cultural settings. Many cultural contexts offer distinctive lenses through which people can comprehend their spirituality and how it affects their mental well-being. We may learn more about how spirituality can improve emotional resilience, offer coping strategies, and create a sense of community by looking at these cultural viewpoints.

1. Native American Spirituality and Nature Connection

As a spiritual practice, indigenous cultures frequently stress having a close relationship with nature. Their worldview is shaped by this interaction, which also lays the groundwork for their emotional stability:

- **Holistic Worldview:** According to many Indigenous beliefs, humans are a part of a broader ecological system and the globe is an interconnected web. Emotional well-being can result from this holistic viewpoint, which encourages respect for all living things and a sense of duty toward the environment.
- **outdoors as Healer:** Spending time in outdoors is revered as a spiritual discipline. Foraging, hunting, and getting together with others in natural environments are examples of activities that can be therapeutic as well as spiritual. The therapeutic advantages of this connection are further supported by research demonstrating how spending time in nature can lower stress, anxiety, and sadness.
- **Rituals and Traditions:** Seasonal celebrations and rites of passage are examples of rituals that are part of Indigenous spiritual practices that celebrate the cycles of nature. Rituals like this provide people a sense of order and community, which promotes emotional stability and cohesiveness.

2. Eastern Thought and Awareness

Spirituality and intellectual teachings, especially those of Buddhism and Hinduism, are entwined in many Eastern cultures:

- **Mindfulness and Meditation:** The core of these ideologies is the practice of mindfulness, which invites people to be conscious of their thoughts and feelings in the moment. Numerous studies have shown that mindfulness meditation improves emotional control, lowers stress, and supports mental health in general.
- **Impermanence:** Eastern spiritual traditions frequently stress how fleeting life is. Comprehending the transient nature of emotions

and circumstances can cultivate adaptability, enabling people to confront obstacles with a more impartial viewpoint.

- **Compassion and Interconnectedness:** These customs encourage compassion toward others as well as toward oneself. This kind perspective encourages communal support and social ties, both of which are essential for mental well-being.

3.   Abrahamic Faiths and Social Assistance

The three Abrahamic religions—Islam, Christianity, and Judaism—offer different but complementary frameworks for spirituality and mental well-being.

- Trust and Faith: A major component of these faiths is trust in a higher power. Through a sense of purpose and confidence in divine wisdom, this faith can promote emotional resilience and provide consolation and hope during trying times.
- Community and Belonging: Social support, which is essential for mental health, is obtained through involvement in religious communities. Common interests and practices, including prayer, worship, and almsgiving, forge links that strengthen emotional fortitude and act as a safety net in times of need.
- Rituals and Practices: Stable and regular routines are fostered by rituals like prayer, fasting, and group get-togethers. These activities provide emotional support in addition to spiritual sustenance.

4.   Western Methodologies and Individual Development

Spirituality has gradually moved in Western contexts to emphasize personal development and self-discovery:

- **Psychological Integration:** In order to promote emotional well-being, modern psychology frequently incorporates spirituality. Spiritual components may be used into cognitive-behavioral therapy and other practices to assist people in reframing their ideas and attitudes in order to build resilience and coping mechanisms.

- **Individualism and Self-Expression:** Individualism is highly valued in Western societies, which permits a wide variety of spiritual activities. By giving people the freedom to select behaviors that are in line with their own experiences and worldviews, this introspective inquiry can improve emotional resilience.
- **Spiritual but Not Religious (SBNR):** This is a developing trend that accepts spirituality outside of formal religion in Western societies. Because it enables people to create their own spiritual experiences, this approach can promote emotional health by enabling a more individualized connection to spirituality.

5. Influences from Across Cultures and Globalization

The modern world's interconnection has made it easier for spiritual traditions to spread between cultures:

- **Hybrid Practices:** A lot of people these days combine aspects of many spiritual traditions to create individualized routines that speak to their varied upbringings. This combination can improve emotional resilience by giving people a more comprehensive toolkit to deal with stress and hardship.
- **Resource Access:** The availability of spiritual resources, such as books, seminars, and online groups, has expanded due to globalization. People can now investigate spiritual practices from many civilizations, which enhances their comprehension of mental well-being.
- **The Sensitivity to Culture:** It is imperative that we approach spirituality with cultural sensitivity as we navigate this global world. Respect for different traditions can be encouraged and appropriation can be avoided by having an understanding of the historical and cultural backgrounds of spiritual activities.

Cultural viewpoints on spirituality and mental health highlight the variety of ways people might overcome obstacles in life and improve their quality of life. Every cultural framework gives important insights into the human experience, from Abrahamic religions' communal support to Indigenous links to environment and Eastern mindfulness philosophies.

We can enhance our personal journeys toward emotional balance by acknowledging and honoring these many spiritual practices. Examine how the spiritual practices presented in this book are influenced by your own cultural background as you study them. Accept the aspects that speak to you and be receptive to the wealth of knowledge found in the diverse range of spiritual traditions. We will explore meditation as a route to inner calm in the upcoming chapter, providing helpful advice for starting a fruitful meditation practice.

In summary

There is a strong and complex relationship between spirituality and emotional health. We can develop resilience, discover meaning in life, and improve our general emotional well-being by investigating and incorporating spiritual practices into our daily routines. Think about how spirituality affects your quest for harmony and tranquility as you examine your own convictions and routines.

We will explore meditation as a means of achieving inner peace in the upcoming chapter, providing helpful guidelines for starting a fruitful meditation practice. Consider your personal spiritual beliefs and how they might guide you on your journey as you get ready for this exploration. Recall that spirituality is a personal path that can lead to both emotional healing and deep discoveries.

Chapter 4

The Healing Power of Prayer

For ages, people of many cultures and faiths have used prayer as a meaningful spiritual practice. It acts as a channel for interaction with the divine, a declaration of hope, and a consoling presence amid trying circumstances. This chapter will look at how prayer can help people feel less stressed and more in control of their emotions. It will also look at various spiritual traditions' approaches to prayer and how to incorporate it into daily life.

The Benefits of Prayer for Stress Reduction

Prayer has a major impact on stress reduction and mental health in a number of ways:

1. **Psychological Comfort**: Praying can assist people in feeling psychologically comfortable. It creates a safe area for people to communicate their desires, fears, and worries. Sharing one's troubles with others can help reduce emotions of hopelessness and loneliness.

2. **Connection to a Higher Power:** The idea that they are a part of something bigger or more purposeful provides comfort to a lot of people. This relationship might give one hope by reassuring them that they are not the only ones going through difficult times. Such a mindset can foster resilience in the face of adversity by reducing feelings of helplessness.

3. **Mindfulness and Focus**: Focusing on the here and now via prayer frequently promotes mindfulness. By diverting attention from stressors and unfavorable ideas and encouraging serenity and clarity, this concentration helps lower anxiety.

4. **Social Support:** Congregational worship or group prayer promotes a feeling of community and belonging. Emotional well-being depends on social support, and praying with others can deepen relationships and offer consolation in common religion.

5. Routine and Stability: Including prayer in everyday activities might help to provide stability and structure. Maintaining this routine might strengthen emotional resilience by offering solace during uncertain or changing situations.

Diverse Spiritual Traditions' Attitudes toward Prayer

Different cultures and religions have different ways of expressing prayer. Gaining insight into these methods can improve your personal prayer life and give you a more nuanced understanding of the efficacy of prayer.

1. Religion: Christianity

- **Prayer Styles**: Christian prayer can take many different forms, such as intercession, supplication, confession, and thankfulness. Every variety fulfills a distinct function, cultivating an all-encompassing connection with the Divine.

- **The Weeping Prayer:** Three major Christian tenets are encapsulated in this prayer: accepting divine sovereignty, expressing thankfulness, and seeking guidance. Saying this prayer might make you feel connected to and at ease.

2. Islam

- **Salah:** One of the major tenets of Islam is the five times a day that Muslims offer prayers (Salah). These planned prayers give times of introspection and spiritual connection with Allah while establishing a pattern in daily life.

- **Dua:** Muslims offer personal supplication, or dua, to convey their needs, wishes, and gratitude outside of the prescribed prayer times. The emotional intimacy with the divine is enhanced by this intimate relationship.

3. Judaism:

- **Ritual and Prayer:** In Judaism, ritual actions like donning a tallit or putting on tefillin are frequently performed in conjunction with prayer. Through the development of a strong sense of connection, these rituals heighten the sacredness of prayer.

- **The Shema and Amidah:** Important prayers such as the Shema highlight God's unity and dedication to religion. The Amidah is a fundamental prayer that incorporates thanksgiving, praising, and requesting, allowing for individual expression within a group setting.

4. Buddhism:

- **Chanting and Mantras:** In Buddhism, reciting mantras is a type of prayer that develops compassion and concentrates the mind. These exercises help improve emotional intelligence and mindfulness.

- **Meditation:** Buddhist prayer frequently places a strong emphasis on meditation, which helps people connect with their inner selves and cultivate acceptance and serenity.

5. Hinduism:

- **Janpa (chanting):** In Hinduism, it is customary to repeat holy words or the names of gods. This repetition can help cultivate a sense of divine connection and mental focus.

- **Puja (Ritual Worship):** Offerings to deities are a common part of Hindu rituals, which combine physical acts of devotion with prayer. The bond between the devotee and the divine is strengthened by this practice.

6. Indigenous Spirituality:

- **Ceremonial Prayer:** Ceremonial prayers honoring the planet, ancestors, and the interdependence of all beings are practiced by many Indigenous societies. These prayers frequently incorporate customs that improve mental health and communal ties.

- **Nature as a Source of Prayer:** Prayer has a close relationship with nature for certain Indigenous peoples. Making offerings, singing, or telling stories to the natural environment is a spiritual practice that promotes emotional well-being.

Including Prayer in Everyday Activities

Including prayer in everyday activities can have a profound impact. The following doable actions can assist you in creating a meaningful prayer routine:

1. **Create a Schedule:** Whether it's in the morning, right before dinner, or right before bed, set aside certain times for prayer. Maintaining consistency fosters the habit and establishes a special area for introspection.

2. **Establish a Sacred Space:** Choose a calm, serene location for prayer. This area can have inspirational pictures, candles, or crystals, among other significant items. During prayer, having a designated area improves intention and focus.

3. **Use Prayer Prompts:** Think about utilizing prompts if you find it difficult to know what to say. Consider certain aspects of your life, such as gratitude, difficulties, and desires, and let your prayers reflect these. You can also make your intentions clear by journaling your thoughts.

4. **Include Meditation:** To enhance your practice, combine meditation and prayer. After some quiet introspection, pray to convey your thanks, ask for wisdom, or show compassion.

5. **Practice Gratitude:** Incorporate gratitude into your prayers. Expressing appreciation for the positive aspects of your life can shift your perspective and enhance emotional well-being.

6. **Engage with Community:** Join a spiritual or religious community to share prayer experiences with others. Group prayer can foster a sense of belonging and amplify the emotional benefits of prayer.

7. **Be Open and Authentic:** Approach prayer with an open heart. Authenticity is key—express your true thoughts and feelings, whether they are filled with joy or laden with struggle. This sincerity can deepen your connection to the divine.

Conclusion

The healing power of prayer is profound, offering comfort, connection, and emotional resilience. By exploring various approaches to prayer across cultures and integrating these practices into daily life, individuals can cultivate a deeper sense of peace and balance. As you reflect on your own relationship with prayer, consider how it can serve as a vital tool in your journey toward emotional well-being.

In the next chapter, we will explore mindfulness and the practice of living in the present moment, offering techniques to enhance awareness and reduce stress. As you prepare for this exploration, take a moment to consider how prayer has played a role in your life and how it might evolve as you seek greater emotional balance.

Chapter 5

Mindfulness: Living in the Present Moment

The practice of mindfulness, which involves being totally present and involved in the here and now without passing judgment, has drawn a lot of attention lately due to its profoundly positive effects on mental well-being. Mindfulness, which has its roots in antiquated spiritual traditions, has been transformed into contemporary activities that improve wellbeing and emotional fortitude. This chapter examines the fundamentals of mindfulness, how it reduces stress, several methods for incorporating mindfulness into daily life, and activities that help you develop your mindfulness practice.

The Mindfulness Principles

The foundational ideas of mindfulness help practitioners develop a present-focused awareness. These principles include:

1. **Awareness:** The capacity to recognize ideas, feelings, and sensations as they arise is the fundamental component of mindfulness. People are encouraged by this awareness to watch their experiences without being overwhelmed or reacting.

2. **Non-Judgment**: Being mindful encourages one to view experiences without passing judgment. Rather than categorizing emotions or thoughts as "good" or "bad," practitioners learn to accept them as a natural aspect of being human. Emotional clarity is promoted and internal conflict is lessened by this acceptance.

3. **Emphasis on the Present Moment**: Mindfulness highlights the significance of the current moment. People can liberate themselves from concerns about the past or the future by focusing their attention on the present, which fosters a sense of stability and serenity.

4. **Curiosity:** Mindfulness is improved by developing a curious mind about one's experiences. Keeping an open mind when dealing with ideas and emotions encourages investigation and a better understanding, which enhances mindfulness practice.

5. **Compassion:** Self- and other-compassion is fostered by mindfulness. By fostering emotional resilience, this compassionate awareness enables people to face obstacles with kindness and understanding.

Mindfulness's Effect on Stress

From Stress to Serenity: Spiritual Techniques for Emotional Balance

Studies have demonstrated that practicing mindfulness can dramatically lower stress and enhance emotional health in general:

1. **Diminished Stress Reactions:** It has been discovered that mindfulness techniques reduce cortisol levels, the hormone linked to stress. People who are less stressed physiologically exhibit fewer emotional and physical symptoms.

2. **Improved Emotional Regulation:** Mindfulness encourages increased emotional awareness, which enables people to react to challenges in a cool, collected manner. This improved emotional control lessens overwhelming and anxious feelings.

3. **Enhanced Clarity and Focus:** Mindfulness enhances cognitive performance, decision-making, and problem-solving skills by teaching the mind to concentrate on the here and now. People are able to approach problems with a more concentrated and innovative perspective thanks to this clarity.

4. **Enhanced Resilience:** Consistent mindfulness practice increases resilience by assisting people in developing a fair-minded outlook on life's obstacles. Practitioners who possess heightened emotional awareness are better equipped to overcome obstacles and overcome failures.

Methods for Bringing Mindfulness into Everyday Tasks

Practicing mindfulness on a regular basis can be easy yet incredibly beneficial. The following are some practical methods for incorporating mindfulness into your daily routine:

1. **Mindful Breathing**: To ground yourself in the here and now, pay attention to your breath. Breathe deeply for a few moments, observing the movement of air entering and exiting your body. If your mind wanders, gently guide it back to your breath.

2. **Body Scan:** This technique entails focusing on various body areas and noting any tightness or sensations. Beginning at your toes and moving up to your head, pause to notice the sensation in each location.

3. **Mindful Eating**: Slow down and appreciate each bite of food to transform mealtime into a mindfulness exercise. Take note of your food's flavors, textures, and fragrances. This technique encourages healthy eating habits in addition to improving the dining experience.

4. **Walking Meditation**: Concentrate on the feelings of each step while you practice walking meditation. As you walk, pay attention to the way your feet hit the ground, how your legs move, and the rhythm of your breath. You can perform this exercise outside or indoors.

5. **Mindful Listening**: When having a discussion, focus entirely on the other person and refrain from planning your reply while they are speaking. This promotes deeper understanding and strengthens your relationships with other people.

6. **Mindfulness in Daily Tasks**: Bring mindfulness to mundane chores like brushing your teeth or doing the dishes. Consider the exercise to be a type of meditation as you pay attention to the movements, sounds, and sensations it involves.

Activities and Practices for Mindfulness

Here are some activities you can do on a daily basis to enhance your mindfulness practice:

1. **Five Senses Exercise**: Use your five senses to ground yourself for a time. Count the following: five objects are visible, four are tactile, three are auditory, two are olfactory, and one is gustatory. This practice improves sensory appreciation and increases awareness of the current moment.

2. **Gratitude Mindfulness**: Take a few minutes every day to consider your blessings. This exercise promotes appreciation for the current moment and positive attitude.

3. **Mindful Journaling:** Set aside time to write in your journal about your feelings and ideas without passing judgment. Journaling is a useful mindfulness exercise that can help you better understand your feelings and become more self-aware.

4. **Guided Meditation:** To learn about mindfulness techniques, use guided meditation applications or videos. These materials, particularly for novices, can offer direction and assistance.

5. **Mindfulness Retreats or Workshops:** To enhance your practice, think about going to a mindfulness retreat or workshop.

Immersion events can provide insightful knowledge and practical methods, as well as chances to meet like-minded people.

In summary

Being mindful is an effective technique that can change how we view life. Mindfulness effectively reduces stress and improves emotional resilience because it promotes acceptance, awareness, and compassion. Recall that mindfulness is a skill that takes patience and practice as you work through the methods and activities in this chapter.

We will explore yoga as a holistic approach to emotional well-being in the next chapter, looking at how this age-old discipline unites the body, mind, and spirit. Think back on your mindfulness experiences as you prepare for this investigation and brainstorm ways to use these techniques to achieve better emotional equilibrium in your everyday life.

Chapter 6

Yoga: Union of Body, Mind, and Spirit

Yoga is a traditional Indian form of exercise that is sometimes referred to as a holistic approach to wellness that unites the body, mind, and soul. Yoga is a system of beliefs and practices that goes beyond physical poses in order to support emotional equilibrium and general well-being. This chapter will cover the advantages of yoga for mental well-being, discuss various yoga types, and offer easy poses that can reduce stress and build emotional fortitude.

The Advantages of Yoga for Mental Well-Being

Many of the advantages that yoga provides can greatly improve emotional well-being:

1. **Reduced Stress:** Yoga encourages relaxation and stimulates the parasympathetic nervous system, which reduces stress. Practitioners can experience a deep sense of relaxation, relieve tension, and lower cortisol levels by concentrating on breath and movement.

2. **Better Emotional Regulation:** Yoga increases body and mind awareness, which helps people identify and manage their emotions more intelligently. This increased self-awareness fosters emotional resilience and aids in the management of challenging emotions.

3. **Improved Mind-Body Connection:** Yoga places a strong emphasis on the relationship between emotional and physical states. People who possess this awareness are able to comprehend how stress physically shows up in their bodies, which makes it easier to treat emotional health holistically.

4. **Mindfulness Promotion:** By incorporating mindfulness principles into their practices, yoga instructors encourage their students to maintain full attention and present-mind awareness while they move. By fostering acceptance and non-judgment, this mindfulness practice helps lessen anxiety and pessimism.

5. **Support and Community:** Taking group yoga courses helps people feel supported and a part of the community. Strong social ties are forged via practice together, and these relationships are essential for resilience and emotional support.

6. **Empowerment and Confidence:** Developing one's yoga practice and mastering positions can help one feel empowered and

accomplished. This increase in self-assurance might have a good effect on one's emotional health and perspective on life.

Various Yoga Styles

There are many different forms of yoga, and each has its own advantages and methods. These are a few of the most well-liked looks:

1. **Hatha Yoga:** With an emphasis on fundamental alignment and poses, Hatha is frequently regarded as the cornerstone style of yoga. It stresses gradual movement, breath control, and relaxation, making it perfect for beginners.

2. **Vinyasa Yoga:** Vinyasa is a dynamic style of yoga that flows through positions in time with the breath. This approach is a great option for people who want to incorporate mindfulness and movement because it encourages both mental and physical wellness.

3. **Yin Yoga:** Yin yoga is a form of yoga that focuses on deep connective tissues through long-held passive positions. This meditation technique is good for releasing emotions and reducing stress since it promotes introspection and relaxation.

4. **Restorative Yoga:** This kind of yoga allows for profound relaxation and healing by supporting the body in soft positions using props. This technique works very well to lower tension and encourage emotional equilibrium.

5. **Ashtanga Yoga:** Ashtanga is an exacting, methodical practice that calls for a predetermined series of poses to be executed in a

particular order. This approach can improve resilience by strengthening mental and physical discipline.

6. **Kundalini Yoga:** Kundalini uses movement, breathing, and chanting to activate spiritual energy. This is a profound option for individuals who are looking for deeper transformation because it attempts to promote both spiritual and emotional healing.

Easy Yoga Asana Practices for Emotional Balance and Stress Reduction

Including yoga in your everyday practice can be easy and beneficial. The following are some easily attainable yoga poses that help reduce stress and encourage emotional equilibrium:

1. **Flow in the Morning (10–15 minutes):**
   - Begin on your hands and knees in the Cat-Cow Pose (Marjaryasana-Bitilasana). Breathe in as you curve your spine (Cat) and out as you arch your back (Cow). Do this five times.
   - Adho Mukha Svanasana (Downward-Facing Dog): Starting on your hands and knees, raise your hips back and up to form an inverted V. Feel the stretch in your legs and spine as you hold for five breaths.
   - Child's Pose (Balasana): Bend forward, sit back on your heels, and stretch your arms out in front of you. Breathe deeply for five breaths while placing your forehead on the mat.

2. **Midday Reset (10–15 minutes):**

Sit with your legs extended in the seated forward bend pose (paschimottanasana). Take a breath, extend your back, and release it as you bend forward. Hold for five breaths, concentrating on tension release.

- Uttanasana (Standing Forward Bend): Place your feet hip-width apart. Fold forward, allowing your head to hang heavily, and hinge at the hips. Take five deep breaths and hold.

- Simple Pose (Sukhasana) with Breathwork: Sit with your legs crossed, close your eyes, and concentrate on your breathing. For four counts, inhale, hold, and then exhale. Continue for five cycles.

3. **Evening Wind-Down (15–20 minutes):**
   - Supta Matsyendrasana, or the supine spinal twist, involves lying on your back, bringing one knee up to the chest, and then slowly twisting it throughout your body. Hold each side for five breaths.

   - **Legs-Up-the-Wall Pose (Viparita Karani):** The pose involves lying on your back and extending your legs up a wall. This little inversion encourages calmness. Breathe deeply while holding for five to ten minutes.

   - **Savasana (Corpse Pose):** Place your arms at your sides and lie flat on your back. Allow your body to completely relax while you close your eyes and concentrate on your breathing. Hold this position for five to ten minutes.

Jake A Waldron

Short Glossary of Yoga Terms for Beginners

1. **Asana:** A yoga stance or physical posture intended to enhance balance, strength, and flexibility.

2. **Pranayama:** Breath control techniques that improve the body's energy flow and encourage concentration and relaxation.

3. **Savasana:** Also referred to as Corpse Pose, this resting pose is usually performed to encourage deep relaxation at the conclusion of a yoga practice.

4. **Namaste:** a customary salutation that means "I bow to you," commonly used as a show of respect at the start or finish of a yoga practice.

5. **Ujjayi Breath:** This deep, oceanic breath is produced by slightly tightening the throat to produce a calming sound. It is frequently utilized in Vinyasa and Ashtanga yoga.

6. **Vinyasa:** This dynamic yoga style flows from one pose to the next by coordinating breath and movement.

7. **Yin Yoga:** This meditative form of yoga targets deep connective tissues and encourages relaxation by having practitioners hold passive positions for prolonged periods of time.

8. **Hatha Yoga:** Suitable for beginners, this basic style of yoga emphasizes physical postures, alignment, and breathwork.

9. **Chaturanga Dandasana:** This pushup pose, which is frequently included in Vinyasa sequences, calls for strong arms and a stable core.

10. **Kundalini:** This kind of yoga uses movement, breathing, and chanting to activate spiritual energy.

11. **Dharma:** In yoga, dharma refers to living in harmony with one's inner self. It also refers to one's purpose or responsibility in life.

12. **Mudra:** In yoga and meditation, hand gestures or seals are used to improve energy flow and support particular aims.

13. **Drishti:** During yoga practice, a focused gaze or center of concentration is employed to enhance balance and mental clarity.

14. **Mantra:** To focus the mind and summon spiritual energy, repeat a sacred word or phrase during meditation or other exercise.

15. **Chakras:** Often mentioned in yoga philosophy, chakras are energy centers in the body that correlate to various physical, emotional, and spiritual aspects of being.

This dictionary helps novices participate with their practice with confidence by giving them a basic comprehension of fundamental yoga terms.

Chapter 7

Breathwork: Harnessing the Power of Your Breath

Breath is a crucial factor that affects our physical, emotional, and spiritual well-being. It is the link between our body and mind. Across nations and traditions, breathwork—a discipline centered on mindful breathing techniques—has been used to improve health, lower stress levels, and promote emotional equilibrium. This chapter will address the role that breathing plays in stress and emotion management, go over a variety of breathwork methods, and offer guided exercises that you can use to start incorporating breathwork into your daily routine.

The Value of Breath in Stress and Emotion Management

Not only is breathing necessary for survival, but it is also an effective technique for controlling our emotional states. The effects of mindful breathing on stress and mental well-being are as follows:

1. **The nerve System Regulation**: Our stress reaction is governed by the autonomic nerve system, which is directly impacted by our breathing. Breathing deeply and slowly triggers the parasympathetic nervous system, which in turn promotes relaxation and lessens the stress-related fight-or-flight response.

2. **Emotional Release**: Shallow or irregular breathing is a common physical sign of the emotional strain that many individuals carry in their bodies. By assisting with the relaxation of this tension, conscious breathwork can promote the expression and release of emotions.

3. **Enhanced Awareness**: Mindfulness and present-moment awareness are fostered by concentrating on the breath. By encouraging people to notice their thoughts and feelings without passing judgment, this technique helps people achieve a more stable emotional state.

4. **Improved Energy Flow**: Breath is frequently regarded as a vital life force, or prana in yoga terminology. The body's energy flows more freely when breathwork is done correctly, which boosts vigor and elevates mood.

5. **Better Clarity and attention**: Deep breathing improves attention and clarity by increasing oxygen flow to the brain. Emotional control and sound decision-making depend on this mental acuity.

Different Breathwork Methods

There are various breathwork methods, and each has special advantages. Here are a few well-liked techniques:

1. Diaphragmatic Breathing, often known as "Belly Breathing," is a breathing method in which the diaphragm is used to breathe deeply instead of the chest. It eases anxiousness and encourages relaxation.
   - Techniques for Practice: Comfortably lie down or sit. Grasp your abdomen with one hand and your chest with the other. Breathe deeply through your nose, letting your chest remain motionless as your belly rises. Feel your tummy drop as you gently release the breath through your mouth. Continue for a few minutes.

2. Box breathing: Also referred to as square breathing, this method is frequently employed to improve concentration and lessen tension.

- o To practice, take a four-count breath, hold it for four counts, exhale for four counts, and then hold it again for four counts. Continue in this manner for a few minutes.

3. Dr. Andrew Weil's 4-7-8 Breathing Method: This method encourages relaxation and lessens anxiety.

   - o To practice, take a quiet breath via your nose for four counts, hold it for seven counts, and then exhale fully through your mouth for eight counts. Four times through, repeat the cycle.

4. Alternate nostril breathing, or nadi shodhana, is a yoga pose that promotes relaxation and clarity by balancing the left and right hemispheres of the brain.

   - o Practice tip: Take a comfortable seat. Close your right nostril with your thumb. Take a deep breath through your left nose. Using your right ring finger, shut the left nostril, open the right one, and release the breath. Breathe in via your right nostril, shut it, then release the air through your left. Continue for multiple iterations.

5. Sitalini Breath, also known as the "Cooling Breath," is a common method for calming the mind and cooling the body.

   - o Practice tip: If you can, sit comfortably and roll your tongue into a tube. Taking a deep breath through your mouth, notice how chilly it feels. Shut your mouth and release the breath via your nose. Simply take a deep breath through your mouth and release it through your nose if you are unable to roll your tongue.

6. Kapalabhati (Skull Shining Breath): a forceful breathing exercise that invigorates and cleanses the internal organs.

o Techniques for Practice: Maintain a straight spine and sit comfortably. Take a deep breath, then push out through your nose while tensing your abdominal muscles. Let your breath come in passively. After 30 to 60 seconds of repetition, resume your regular breathing.

Assisted Activities to Include Breathwork in Everyday Activities

Stress can be decreased and emotional equilibrium can be improved by incorporating breathwork into daily life. To get you going, try these guided exercises:

1. **Morning Breath Ritual (5–10 minutes):** 1. Take a seat comfortably.
   - Start by employing diaphragmatic breathing, paying attention to long, slow breaths.
   - Make the five cycles of Box Breathing transition.
   - Finish by taking a few quiet moments to contemplate and make a plan for the rest of the day.

2. **Stress-Relief Break (3-5 minutes):**
   - Every time you feel anxious, stop and breathe.
   - To help you relax, practice 4-7-8 Breathing for multiple cycles.
   - Get back to your tasks with a sense of clarity and renewal.

3. **Evening Wind-Down (10 minutes):**
   - Find a comfortable place to sit or lie down.
   - To balance your energy, do five minutes of Nadi Shodhana.
   - Conclude with a Sitali Breath to encourage calm and get ready for bed.

4. **Breath Awareness Throughout the Day:** Make notes to check in with your breath on your calendar or phone throughout the day.

    ○ Whenever you feel tension rising, take a moment to stop, pay attention to your breathing, and practice diaphragmatic breathing.

Breath of the Day: A Morning Routine to Promote Wellness

We present the "Breath of the Day" concept to help you include breathwork into your regular routine. You can practice a certain breathing method every day to improve your emotional balance, increase awareness, and lower stress levels. How to apply this exercise in your daily life is as follows:

How to Perform the "Daily Breath"

1. Select Your Breath: Choose one breathing method to concentrate on at the start of each day. You can pick a technique that best suits your needs or current emotional state, or you can go through the strategies presented in this chapter in order of introduction.
2. Decide on a Time: Set aside a certain amount of time every day for your "Breath of the Day" routine. This might be done in the afternoon to rejuvenate, in the morning to establish a positive tone, or in the evening to decompress.
4. Establish a Ritual: Look for a calm area where you can practice without discomfort. To improve the atmosphere, you may apply essential oils, play some relaxing music, or light a candle. Making a ritual can assist your body and mind know when it's time to practice concentrated breathing.
5. Length: Make time to practice your selected breathing technique for a minimum of five to ten minutes. You can prolong this period for more profound awareness and relaxation if time permits.
6. Reflect: After practicing, pause to consider your feelings. Take note of any alterations in your mental clarity, feelings, or bodily experiences. To monitor your development and insights over time, think about keeping a journal of your reflections.
7. Share Your Experience: If it makes you feel better, tell your friends, family, or the yoga community about your "Breath of the Day" experience. Everyone involved may benefit from this sharing's ability to promote accountability and build a positive environment.

Techniques for "Breath of the Day" Example

- o **Monday: Diaphragmatic Breathing**
  To encourage grounding and relaxation, concentrate on taking deep belly breaths.
- **Tuesday: Box Breathing**
  Apply this method to improve relaxation and concentrate, particularly before difficult tasks.
- **Wednesday: 4–7 Breathing**
  Use this method to reduce anxiety and get ready for a good night's sleep.
- **Thursday: Nadi Shodhana**
  Use alternate nostril breathing to maintain a balance of energy and mental clarity.
- **Friday: Sitali Breath**
  Remain cool and collected, particularly following a demanding workweek.
- **Saturday: Kapalabhati**
  Use this energizing method to energize your body and erase mental cobwebs.
- **Sunday:** Incorporate thankfulness into your routine by taking a moment to breathe consciously and reflect on your week.

A straightforward yet effective technique to develop a stronger bond with your breath and mental health is to adopt the "Breath of the Day" concept. You may cultivate mindfulness, strengthen your emotional well-being, and become more resilient to stress by setting aside time each day to concentrate on your breathing. Breathwork will become a vital tool in your toolbox for balance and tranquility as you go on this daily journey.

We will delve into the transformational power of affirmations and thankfulness in the upcoming chapter, learning how these practices can further improve your everyday life and emotional well-being. In preparation for this next exploration, consider how your breath practices are impacting your journey.

In summary

Breathwork is a potent technique that promotes awareness, calm, and resilience and has the potential to completely change your emotional well-being. You may develop more calm and wellbeing in your life by learning to use the power of your breath. As you experiment with different methods and incorporate breathwork into your daily routine, consider how this exercise improves emotional equilibrium and facilitates your transition from stress to calm.

We will explore the importance of affirmations and thankfulness in the upcoming chapter, as well as how these practices might improve emotional well-being even further. Think about how aware breathing has changed your life and how it might be a tool for more emotional clarity and resilience as you get ready for this inquiry.

Chapter 9

The Role of Gratitude and Affirmations

Affirmations and gratitude are effective strategies for improving mental health and cultivating optimism. Both techniques promote perspective shifting, which enables people to build resilience in the face of adversity and concentrate on the good things in life. This chapter delves into the science of affirmations, the power of gratitude practices to improve emotional wellness, and useful strategies for implementing both into your everyday life.

How Practicing Gratitude Can Improve Emotional Health

Being grateful is a habit that can have a big impact on mental health and emotional stability; it's not just a passing emotion. The following are some ways that practicing thankfulness might improve emotional health:

1. **Reorients Attention from Negativity to Positivity**: Expressing gratitude helps people recognize and value the good things in their lives, which can offset negative thought patterns. This change in perspective might enhance contentment and outlook in general.

2. **Strengthens Resilience**: Expressing gratitude on a regular basis fosters emotional resilience. Acknowledging good experiences makes people more resilient to stress and hardship, building a wall against emotional difficulties.

3. **Strengthens Relationships**: By encouraging connection and reciprocal appreciation, expressing thankfulness can improve relationships. People who express their gratitude to others build stronger relationships by creating a positive feedback loop.

4. **Enhances Mental Health**: Studies have indicated that cultivating appreciation can lessen anxiety and depressive symptoms. People can feel more purposeful and have a higher level of life satisfaction when they concentrate on the positive aspects of life.

5. **Encourages Mindfulness**: Gratitude forces people to consider and value their current circumstances, which promotes mindfulness. This practice of mindfulness can improve emotional clarity and lower stress.

Making and Applying Affirmations to Maintain Emotional Equilibrium

Positive statements known as affirmations can upend negative thought patterns and bolster optimism and self-worth. They may be very important in fostering emotional equilibrium:

1. **Reinforcement of Positive Beliefs**: By reiterating positive beliefs about oneself and one's situation, affirmations assist in combating negative self-talk. Affirmations can be repeatedly repeated to help people change the way they talk to themselves.

2. **Boosting Self-Esteem**: Affirmations have the power to increase confidence and self-worth. People who hear positive affirmations are more empowered because they are inspired to acknowledge their own abilities and strengths.

3. **Focus on Goals and Intentions**: Affirmations can serve as reminders of personal goals and intentions, helping individuals stay motivated and aligned with their aspirations. This focus can enhance a sense of purpose and direction in life.

4. **Reduction of Stress and Anxiety**: By replacing negative thoughts with positive affirmations, individuals can reduce feelings of stress and anxiety. Affirmations promote a more optimistic outlook, which can alleviate emotional burdens.

Practical Tips for Incorporating Gratitude and Affirmations into Daily Life

Incorporating gratitude and affirmations into your daily routine can be simple and rewarding. The following are tips to help you start:

1. **Gratitude Journaling**: - Set aside time each day to write down three to five things you are grateful for. This practice helps solidify positive experiences and encourages reflection on the good in your life.
   o Consider varying your entries by focusing on different aspects of life, such as relationships, experiences, or personal strengths.
2. **Daily Affirmation Practice:** - Choose a set of affirmations that resonate with you and reflect your goals or values. Write them down and repeat them aloud daily, preferably in front of a mirror.
   o Affirmations can be tailored to specific areas of your life, such as self-esteem, health, or career aspirations.

Gratitude Reminders:

Place sticky notes with gratitude prompts around your living space (e.g., on your mirror, fridge, or workspace). These reminders can prompt you to reflect on what you are thankful for throughout the day.

Express Gratitude to Others:

Always express gratitude. Make it a habit. Write thank-you notes, send appreciative texts, or verbally acknowledge the support and kindness you receive.

Create a Gratitude Jar:

Use a jar to collect notes of gratitude. Each time you feel thankful for something, write it down on a slip of paper and add it to the jar. Review the notes periodically to reflect on the abundance in your life.

Combine Practices:

Integrate gratitude and affirmations by creating affirmations based on your gratitude entries. For example, if you're grateful for your supportive friends, an affirmation could be, "I am surrounded by love and support."

Mindful Gratitude Practice: Spend a few minutes each day in mindfulness meditation, focusing on the things you are grateful for. This practice can deepen your appreciation and cultivate a sense of peace.

30-Day Gratitude Challenge

Embarking on a 30-day gratitude challenge can be a transformative way to cultivate a more positive mindset and deepen your appreciation for life. Each day, you'll receive a specific prompt to guide your reflections. Here's the challenge:

Week 1: Gratitude for People

- o **Day 1:** Write about someone who has positively influenced your life and what you appreciate about them.
- o **Day 2:** List three qualities in a friend that you are grateful for and why they matter to you.
- o **Day 3:** Reflect on a family member you're thankful for. Describe a specific memory that makes you smile.
- o **Day 4:** Write a thank-you note (it can be sent or just written for yourself) to someone who has helped you recently.

- o **Day 5:** Think of a mentor or teacher who has inspired you. Write about what you learned from them.
- o **Day 6:** Acknowledge a stranger who made your day better (e.g., a kind cashier or a helpful colleague).
- o **Day 7:** Reflect on a difficult relationship in your life and identify one lesson you learned from it.

Week 2: Gratitude for Experiences

- o **Day 8:** Write about a memorable trip or vacation that brought you joy.
- o **Day 9:** Reflect on a recent challenge you faced and identify what you learned or gained from it.
- o **Day 10:** Describe a small daily routine or ritual that you appreciate (like your morning coffee or evening walks).
- o **Day 11:** Think of a book or movie that impacted you. Write about what you learned or felt.
- o **Day 12:** Write about a hobby or activity that brings you happiness and why you're grateful for it.
- o **Day 13:** Reflect on a moment of silence or stillness that allowed you to connect with your thoughts.
- o **Day 14:** Acknowledge a time when you helped someone else. Reflect on how it made you feel.

Week 3: Gratitude for Nature and Surroundings

- o **Day 15:** Write about a natural setting (park, beach, forest) that you love and why it brings you peace.

o   **Day 16:** Reflect on a favorite season. What do you appreciate most about it?

o   **Day 17:** List three things in your home that make you feel safe and comfortable.

o   **Day 18:** Describe a beautiful sunset or sunrise you witnessed recently. How did it make you feel?

o   **Day 19:** Write about a favorite plant or flower and why it brings you joy.

o   **Day 20:** Reflect on the sounds of nature (birds, waves, rustling leaves) that you appreciate.

o   **Day 21:** Think of a childhood outdoor activity that brought you joy. Write about that memory.

Week 4: Gratitude for Personal Growth

o   **Day 22:** Write about a personal strength that you appreciate in yourself.

o   **Day 23:** Reflect on a recent accomplishment, big or small, and what it means to you.

o   **Day 24:** Describe a fear you've faced and how overcoming it has changed you.

o   **Day 25:** Write about a lesson learned from a failure or setback.

o   **Day 26:** Think of a time when you stepped outside your comfort zone. What did you gain from the experience?

o   **Day 27:** Reflect on your values and write about one that you hold dear. Why is it important to you?

- o **Day 28:** Write a letter to your future self, expressing gratitude for the growth you hope to achieve.

Week 5: Gratitude for the Present and Future

- o **Day 29:** Reflect on three things you are grateful for today, focusing on the present moment.
- o **Day 30:** Write about your hopes and dreams for the future, and express gratitude for the journey ahead.

At the end of this 30-day gratitude challenge, take some time to review your entries. Reflect on the themes that emerged and how your perspective on gratitude has shifted. Consider continuing the practice beyond these 30 days, whether through journaling, sharing with others, or incorporating gratitude into your daily routine. Enjoy the journey!

Conclusion

Gratitude and affirmations are potent practices that can profoundly influence emotional health and resilience. By consciously cultivating gratitude and affirming positive beliefs, individuals can transform their emotional landscape, enhancing their ability to cope with stress and navigate life's challenges.

As you explore the practices of gratitude and affirmations, consider how they can complement the other spiritual techniques discussed in this book. In the next chapter, we will delve into spiritual rituals for stress reduction, discovering how these practices can further enhance your journey from stress to serenity. Reflect on your experiences with gratitude and affirmations as you prepare for this next exploration.

Chapter 9

Spiritual Rituals for Stress Reduction

In spiritual practice, rituals are very important because they provide a disciplined approach to develop awareness, emotional equilibrium, and a connection with the divine. This chapter discusses the value of rituals in spiritual practice, offers several illustrations of spiritual rituals for emotional healing, and offers suggestions for developing stress-reduction practices of one's own.

Rituals' Significance in Spiritual Practice

Rituals are effective means of bringing our emotional states into balance, centering, and grounding. Rituals are important in spiritual practice for the following reasons:

1. Establishes Structure and Routine: Rituals give our lives a feeling of predictability and order. This structure helps establish a safe area for connection and reflection, which may be especially beneficial during stressful times.

2. Promotes Mindfulness: Following routines helps one become more mindful of the current moment. Many rituals' repeating elements help people concentrate, which lowers distractions and fosters a stronger bond between the self and the cosmos.

3. Promotes Connection: Rituals frequently entail shared experiences and a sense of community, which helps to reinforce ties between participants. In stressful situations, this sense of connection can strengthen feelings of support and belonging.

4. Promotes Emotional Release: A lot of rituals incorporate expressive components like storytelling, dancing, or chanting. These features can help people let go of their emotions and digest their experiences in a secure setting.

5. Strengthens Spiritual Bond: Rituals can strengthen a person's spiritual practice by giving them a clear channel to the divine or a higher purpose in life. In the midst of upheaval, this connection can provide solace and calm.

Spiritual Rituals Examples for Emotional Recovery

1. **Lighting of the Candle:**

- Goal: To represent light, hope, and establishing intentions.

- Exercise: While keeping a clear intention in your heart, light a candle in a peaceful area. Imagine the light driving out the negativity and darkness in your life as the flame burns. As you concentrate on your goal, you can say a prayer or recite a mantra.

2. Gratitude Ritual: Goal: To foster appreciation and refocus attention from stress to the good.

- Make time every week to jot down the things you are thankful for. While you reflect, you can play soothing music or light incense. Think about expressing your gratitude to others in writing or vocally.

3. **The Ritual of the Nature Walk:**

- Goal: To foster emotional health and reestablish a connection with nature.

- Exercise: Pick a natural area and deliberately stroll across it. As you stroll, pay attention to your breathing, take in the beauty all around you, and express thankfulness for it all. Give yourself permission to enjoy the experience completely.

4. **Singing or chanting:**

- Goal: To let go of feelings and establish a spiritual energy connection.

- Practice: Pick a song or phrase that makes you feel good. Make time to sing or chant, by yourself or with others. Allow the words and the vibrations of your voice to fill you with awe and uplift your spirits.

5. **Establishing a Sacred Space: -** Goal: To create a physical space devoted to introspection and mindfulness.

- Exercise: Set aside a corner of your house as a place of worship. Adorn it with sentimental objects (such as crystals, pictures, or keepsakes) and utilize it for journaling, prayer, or meditation. Regularly spend time there to develop a peaceful mindset.

6. Ritual Bath: - Intention: To purify and revitalize the body and soul.

- Exercise: Set up a warm bath with plants that speak to you, aromatic oils, or Epsom salts. Imagine that tension and negativity are being washed away by the water while you soak. As you unwind, spend some time in meditation or reflection.

7. The purpose of the full moon or new moon ritual is to set intentions and respect natural cycles.

- **Practice:** Think about what you want to let go of during the full moon, and make plans for the upcoming cycle during the new moon. As a reminder, put your intentions in writing and keep them wherever you can see them.

Establishing Individual Rituals to Control Stress

Making your own rituals might help you deal with stress in a way that suits your particular spiritual path. The following actions can assist you in creating successful personal rituals:

1. **Determine Your Goals**: -Think about the goals you have for your ritual. Is it a stronger spiritual connection, emotional healing, or stress relief? Your intentions will determine the direction of the ritual.

2. **Pick Meaningful Elements:** - Take into account adding components that have special meaning for you. This could include particular hues, smells, designs, or sounds that uplift your mood and improve your experience.

3. **Create a Routine:** - Choose a consistent day and hour for your ritual. Maintaining consistency facilitates the practice's integration into daily life and serves to reinforce it.

4. **Include Mindfulness**: - Give your routine your whole attention throughout. By being conscious of your thoughts, feelings, and bodily sensations, you can cultivate mindfulness. This emphasis will increase the ritual's efficacy.

5. **Permit Flexibility:** Although routines can offer structure, be willing to modify your ritual as circumstances dictate. As you grow as a person and as your life changes, you might eventually adjust your practices.

6. **Consider the Experience:** - After doing each ritual, consider the emotional impact it had on you. To record your experiences, realizations, and any shifts in your emotions or stress levels, think about maintaining a notebook.

7. **Discuss Your Rituals**: Talk to friends or family about your rituals if it makes you feel comfortable. This has the potential to

strengthen your bonds with people who are traveling similar paths and foster a feeling of community.

In summary

Spiritual practices are effective strategies for reducing stress and promoting emotional equilibrium. People can develop a stronger connection to themselves, their emotions, and the world around them by partaking in meaningful activities. Examine the rituals that speak to you and how they might help you transition from tension to calm.

We will examine the rejuvenating effects of spending time in nature in the upcoming chapter, as well as how it may be a source of strength. As you get ready for this next excursion, think back on the rituals you've found and how they might enhance your entire spiritual practice.

Chapter 10:

Connecting with Nature

An excellent source of emotional balance, healing, and grounding is the natural world. The benefits of spending time in nature for mental health, the techniques that can help you connect with the outdoors, and the healing power of nature are all covered in this chapter. Through interacting with your surroundings, you can improve your spiritual practice and discover calm in the middle of life's challenges.

Nature's Healing Power

Nature is naturally calming and healing, offering a haven from the stresses of contemporary life. The following are some main arguments in favor of the emotional health benefits of spending time in nature:

1. Lessens Stress and Anxiety: o Several studies have demonstrated that being in nature reduces levels of cortisol, the hormone linked to stress. People can unwind and revitalize themselves thanks to the relaxing influence of natural surroundings, which helps to reduce anxiety.
2. Improves Mood: Research has connected better mental and emotional wellness with nature. The neurotransmitter serotonin, which is linked to emotions of happiness, is produced in greater amounts when exposed to natural environments. Walking in a park or relaxing by a river are examples of peaceful and uplifted activities.
3. Encourages Mindfulness: o Spending time in nature cultivates awareness of the present moment. We are invited to completely engage our senses by the sights, sounds, and fragrances of the outdoors, which fosters mindfulness and increases our awareness of our thoughts and feelings.
4. Promotes Connection: o Nature encourages a feeling of connectedness, not just with the surroundings but also with ourselves and other people. We can gain a deeper understanding of life's connectivity and a feeling of belonging to something bigger when we spend time outside.

5. Promotes Physical Activity: Taking part in outdoor pursuits like riding, hiking, or gardening enhances physical health, which is strongly associated with mental health. Endorphins, which are released when you exercise, elevate your mood and lessen tension.

Techniques to Include Nature in Your Spiritual Routines

Take into consideration implementing the following routines to tap into the restorative potential of nature:

1. **Shinrin-yoku, or forest bathing:**
   - What It Is: a custom from Japan that entails submerging oneself in a forest.
   - Techniques for Practice: Go on a leisurely stroll through a forest and use all of your senses. Take note of the sights, sounds, and smells surrounding you. Give yourself permission to take deep breaths and feel the peace of the trees.

2. **Walking Meditations:**
   - What It Is: A type of meditation that incorporates awareness and walking.
   - How to Practice: Pick a peaceful outdoor area. Take your time and walk mindfully, paying attention to how your feet feel on the earth. Breathe in rhythm with your movements, focus only on the now, and let go of other distractions.

3. **Nature Journaling:**
   - What It Is: Putting your ideas and emotions about nature in writing or drawing.
   - Practice tip: Take a journal outside in a natural environment. While you're out in the great outdoors, write down your thoughts, feelings, and observations. By doing this, you can improve your mindfulness and strengthen your bond with the natural world.

4. **Gardening:**

- o What It Is: Growing flowers or plants as a means of fostering a relationship with the land.
- o How to Practice: Establish a tiny garden, either in your balcony or backyard using potted plants. Taking care of plants cultivates a feeling of accountability and a bond with the environment.

5. **Mindful Observation:**
   - o What It Is: Devoting time to scrutinize and value the subtleties found in nature.
   - o Practice tip: Go outside and just observe for a while. Concentrate on a single detail, like the way the clouds move or the texture of the leaves. Give yourself permission to observe everything in the now.

6. Nature Rituals:
   - o What It Is: Developing deliberate rituals that use natural components.
   - o How to Practice: Create a nature-based personal routine. This could include gathering natural objects (leaves or stones) and making an altar out of them or utilizing them in meditation. Celebrate the next seasons with a ceremony that shows your appreciation for the bounty of nature.

The Advantages of Outdoor Activities for Mental Health

There are more benefits to spending time in nature than just reducing stress right away. The following are some advantages of being outside over time:

1. **Enhanced Cognitive Function**: Studies show that spending time in nature improves creativity and cognitive capacities. Natural settings can help people focus better and solve problems more adeptly since they excite the brain.
2. **Increased Emotional Resilience**: o Spending time in nature on a regular basis increases emotional resilience. People may recover

from stress and handle life's obstacles better when they are in peaceful, beautiful environments.

3. **A Stronger Sense of Community**: Taking part in outdoor activities that promote social relationships and a sense of belonging, like group treks or community gardening, is beneficial. These connections can improve general wellbeing and offer emotional support.

4. **Improved Spiritual Connection**: o Spiritual inquiry is frequently facilitated by nature. One's sense of spirituality and connectedness to the cosmos might be strengthened by encountering natural wonders like the tranquility of a forest or the beauty of a sunset.

5. **Raised Environmental Awareness**: o Exposure to the natural world can cultivate a sense of environmental responsibility. This knowledge can inspire good deeds that support ecological health, which raises one's sense of purpose and fulfillment in life.

Here are some particular places and things to do that encourage a close bond with nature:

Here are some particular places and things to do that encourage a close bond with nature:

Places

1. National Parks: Yosemite National Park (California, USA) is one example of a park that offers breathtaking scenery, hiking routes, and chances to observe wildlife.
   - o Activity: Trekking to Vernal Fall along the Mist Trail.

2. Botanical Gardens: Kew Gardens in London, UK, for instance, has a stunning assortment of plants from all over the world that are ideal for leisurely strolls and introspective moments.
   - o Activity: Take part in workshops on plant care or guided garden tours.

3. Beaches: o One such location is Laguna Beach in California, USA. It's a calm beach with room for swimming, tanning, and beachcombing.

o   Exercise: Take a beach yoga class or meditate at dawn.

4. Forests:
    o   For instance, California's Redwood National and State Parks are home to towering redwoods and luxuriant undergrowth, making them perfect for fully immersive forest experiences.
    o   Adventure: Take a guided forest bathing excursion.

5. Lakes and Rivers:
    o   One such lake is Lake Louise in Alberta, Canada. It's a gorgeous lake with mountains all around it that's ideal for hiking and kayaking.
    o   Activity: Take a canoe or kayak rental and discover the beauty of the lake.

6. Wildlife Reserves:
    o   One such reserve is Florida's Everglades National Park, which is home to a variety of wildlife and offers a unique habitat ideal for exploration and teaching.
    o   Activity: See alligators and other animals by going on a guided airboat excursion.

7. Hills and Mountains: The Blue Ridge Parkway in North Carolina and Virginia, USA, for instance, provides breathtaking vistas, hiking paths, and picturesque overlooks.
    o   Activity: Take a picnic at a picturesque viewpoint while driving the parkway.

8. Local Parks: o Central Park in New York City, USA, for instance, is an urban garden with lakes, strolling trails, and gardens.
    o   Activity: Go on a nature walk or sign up for a free outdoor yoga class.

Actions

1. Nature Walks:
   - Plan frequent strolls around nearby parks or natural areas. Observe your surroundings as you bring mindfulness into focus.
2. Birdwatching:
   - To identify local bird species, carry binoculars and a field guide. This can be a soothing exercise that raises ecological consciousness.
3. photos:
   - Use photos to convey the splendor of nature. This promotes awareness of the small things in your surroundings and cultivates mindfulness.
4. Nature Journaling:
   - Write or draw in a journal while you're outside. Keep a journal of your thoughts and feelings as you spend time in nature.
5. Gardening:
   - Plant potted plants or make a tiny garden in your backyard. Taking care of plants strengthens one's bond with the soil.
6. Camping:
   - Stay in a natural environment for one or more nights. Take a step back from technology and take in the sights and sounds of nature.
7. Stargazing:
   - To view the night sky, locate a dimly lit spot away from city lights. To identify planets and constellations, use a stargazing app.
8. Nature Retreats:
   - Go on a weekend retreat that emphasizes wellness, mindfulness, or the outdoors. These retreats frequently incorporate meditation exercises and supervised activities.
9. Mindful Eating Outside:

- o Put together a picnic and savor it in a beautiful setting. Savor the tastes and textures of your meal while you take in your environment.
10. Offer Your Time to Conservation Projects:
    - o Participate in neighborhood conservation projects like habitat restoration or tree planting. This strengthens your bond with the land and helps to preserve it.

By encouraging emotional equilibrium and spiritual development, these places and activities can assist you in strengthening your bond with the natural world. Interacting with the natural environment may be a potent source of healing, regardless of your preference for the peace and quiet of a forest or the vibrant colors of a botanical garden.

In summary

There are several advantages of connecting with nature for spiritual development and emotional equilibrium. You can harness the healing power of the natural world and find calm despite life's challenges by adopting outdoor practices into your routine. As you investigate the different methods of connecting with nature, think about how these activities can enhance your overall process of transforming tension into calm.

We shall talk about the significance of creating a caring spiritual community in the upcoming chapter. Interacting with people who are traveling a similar path to you can improve the experience by offering motivation, support, and a stronger feeling of community. Think back on your encounters with nature as you

Chapter 11

Building a Supportive Spiritual Community

A strong spiritual group greatly aids emotional stability and personal development. This chapter will cover the importance of community in spiritual practice, strategies for establishing and maintaining spiritual connections, and ways to interact with online and offline communities.

Community's Significance for Spiritual and Emotional Health

1. **Comparable Experience:**
   - Spiritual groups offer a forum for people to discuss their difficulties, convictions, and experiences. This mutual comprehension fosters a feeling of belonging, which is essential for mental well-being.

2. **Mutual Support:**
   - Having a community around you provides emotional support when things are tough. Members can support, encourage, and share resources with one another, which helps to lessen feelings of loneliness.

3. Collaborative Learning:

- o Spiritual communities support growth and collaborative learning. Interacting with others enables people to investigate alternative viewpoints, enhance their comprehension of spirituality, and uncover novel practices.

4. Accountability and Motivation:

- o Staying involved in spiritual activities can be made more motivating by a sense of community. Members can encourage a sense of dedication and commitment by holding one another accountable and celebrating accomplishments.

5. Opportunities for Service:

- o A lot of spiritual groups take part in outreach and service, giving its members chances to make a positive impact on society. Serving others can strengthen a person's sense of connection and purpose.

6. Rituals and festivities:

- o To commemorate important occasions and turning points in the community, rituals and festivities are frequently held. A stronger sense of joy and connection is fostered by these shared experiences.

Identifying and Nurturing Spiritual Support Networks

1. Determine Your Values and Interests:

- o Consider your interests, values, and spiritual beliefs. Finding a community that supports your wants and aspirations will be made easier if you know what makes you feel good.

2. Investigate Local Options:

- o Look for community organizations, meditation centers, yoga studios, or spiritual or religious groups in your area. Go to free events or workshops to connect with people who share your interests.

3. **Make Use of Online Resources:**
   - o There are a lot of online spiritual communities in the modern digital era. Look through social media sites like Meetup, Facebook, and specialist forums to locate groups that share your interests.

4. **Attend Workshops and Retreats:**
   - o Taking part in seminars, workshops, or retreats can help you develop your spiritual practice and build relationships with others. These gatherings frequently draw people looking for a sense of belonging.

5. **Volunteer:**
   - o Participating in outreach or community service initiatives might introduce you to people who are as dedicated to having a positive impact as you are. Serving the community can be a great way to strengthen ties with other residents.

6. **Be Approachable and Open:**
   - o Approach discussions at community gatherings with interest and openness. Building relationships requires being open to listening to others and sharing your own experiences.

7. **Form Your Organization:**
   - o Consider forming your group if you're having trouble finding others who share your ideals. Taking the lead can draw like-minded people to your book club, meditation group, or spiritual discussion circle, among other groups.

Methods for Interacting with a Spiritual Group

1. **Take Part in Group Practices:**
   - Attend discussion groups, yoga classes, meditation classes, or prayer groups together. Participating in common activities strengthens bonds and promotes a feeling of community.

2. **Share Your Journey:**
   - Talk candidly with your community about the spiritual path you've taken. Relationships can be strengthened and others might be inspired by sharing your struggles, victories, and insights.

3. **Plan Events:**
   - Show initiative by planning get-togethers like potlucks, seminars, or getaways. This has the potential to strengthen bonds within the community and promote unity.

4. **Establish Virtual Connections:**
   - Participate in virtual get-togethers, forums, and social media to interact with online communities. Ask questions, offer your insights, and encourage others as they travel.

5. **Attend Spiritual Retreats:**
   - Take part in retreats that emphasize on one's community and one's own spiritual development. These all-encompassing encounters have the power to strengthen your spiritual practice and create enduring bonds.

6. **Offer Your Skills:**
   - If you are gifted in any particular area, think about sharing them with the community. Volunteering your time, organizing a workshop, or teaching a class can help you build stronger relationships with other people.

7. **Create Accountability Partners**:
   - o Make a connection with a member of your community to act as a partner in accountability. Frequent check-ins can encourage you to stick with your spiritual routines and objectives.

8. **Celebrate Together:**
   - o Take part in group celebrations of significant life events, such birthdays, anniversaries, or seasonal holidays. These happy moments can strengthen the bond between people and the shared experience.

Ways to Engage in Online Communities, especially for Those Who May Be Isolated

Participating in virtual communities can be a rewarding approach to make new friends, particularly for individuals who might otherwise feel alone. The following are some practical strategies for engaging and establishing deep connections in virtual environments:

1. **Sign up for certain forums and groups**
   - o Locate Specialty Communities: Seek out social media groups or forums devoted to particular hobbies or spiritual practices. Discussion and support groups can be found on websites such as Reddit, Facebook Groups, or niche forums.
   - o Take an Active Role: Take part in conversations, offer your opinions, and reply to other people's posts. Participating actively can make you feel more bonded.

2. **Participate in Virtual Workshops and Webinars**
   - o Look Through Online Events: A lot of organizations provide webinars, classes, and virtual workshops on a range of spiritual subjects. By taking part, you can meet people who share your interests and have the opportunity to learn new things.

o   Network During Events: Make introductions and establish connections with other attendees by using chat features or breakout spaces.

3.   **Take part in video sessions or live streaming.**

o   Attend Live Prayer or Meditation Sessions: A lot of spiritual communities and leaders broadcast these events live. Engaging in these can foster a feeling of community.

o   Share Your Own Live Content: If it makes you feel comfortable, think about facilitating a live Q&A session, meditation, or conversation to foster community.

4.   **Make Use of Social Media Sites**
o   Follow Spiritual Influencers: Interact with content on Twitter, TikTok, Instagram, and other platforms from spiritual influencers or leaders. Leaving thoughtful comments on their posts might start important discussions.
o   Establish a Spiritual Page or Profile and share your practices, reflections, and journey. Connecting with followers will help you grow your following. 5. Take Part in Online Challenges: Join 30-Day Challenges that focus on gratitude, mindfulness, or spiritual practices. These challenges are held in many areas. By taking part, you can share your progress and establish connections with others.
o   Use Hashtags: On social media, look for and connect with people taking on similar tasks by using relevant hashtags.

5.   **Participate in Group Initiatives**
o   Work Together on Initiatives: Seek for chances to participate in collective endeavors like writing, collaborative art, or community service. Collaborating creates a sense of unity and connection.

6. **Form or Enroll in an Online Book Club**
   - o Choose Self-Help or Spiritual Books: Spirituality-related reading and discussion can strengthen bonds and spark enlightening debates.
   - o Arrange Regular Meetings: Over time, connections can be developed with the support of regularly scheduled conversations.

7. **Establish Communication with Accountability Partners**
   - o Partner Up: Look for opportunities to serve as an accountability partner in the community or volunteer to do so. Frequent check-ins can foster a supportive relationship and increase motivation.

8. **Talk About Your Thoughts and Experiences**
   - o Share Your Personal Stories: By opening up about your struggles, victories, and spiritual journey, you can inspire and motivate others to do the same.
   - o Write Blog Posts or Articles: To share your knowledge and encourage conversation, think about writing for local blogs or your own website.

9. **Take Part in Virtual Retreats:**
   - o A lot of organizations currently provide online retreats with a mindfulness, spirituality, or personal development theme. Participant connections can grow deeply as a result of these immersive experiences.
   - o Participate in Group Activities: Use the retreat's group conversations and activities to strengthen your relationships with others.

10. **Use Messaging Apps**
   - o Join Group Chats: On services like Discord or WhatsApp, several communities have created special chat groups. These might be quite helpful for continuing discussions and assistance.

  o Establish One-on-One Connections: Don't be afraid to initiate personal talks with people in order to gradually forge deeper bonds.

11. Show transparency and sincerity

  o Admit Your Weaknesses: Being genuine can draw others in. By being honest with others about your thoughts, emotions, and experiences, you can build stronger bonds with them.

  o Be Nice to Others: Providing empathy, encouragement, and support can help to reinforce ties within the community.

In particular, for people who feel alone, participating in online forums offers a priceless chance to make connections with others. It is possible to create sustaining relationships that advance your spiritual development if you actively participate and look for meaningful interactions. Keep in mind that connection is the foundation of community; regardless of distance, your willingness to participate and share can help others feel like they belong.

In summary

Creating a caring spiritual community is crucial for achieving emotional equilibrium and personal development. Making connections with people who are on similar paths can provide you with motivation, support, and a feeling of community. As you look for methods to strengthen these bonds, keep in mind that community is about more than just belonging to a group—it's about developing deep ties that encourage and empower one another.

We shall share personal transformation tales in the last chapter from people who turned to spiritual activities for peace of mind. Their experiences will inspire and enlighten us, serving as a reminder that the road from stress to calm is a common and individual one. As we proceed toward this final exploration, think back on your experiences with community and how these relationships might enhance your spiritual path.

Chapter 12

Personal Stories of Transformation

This chapter will examine first-hand accounts from people who have used different spiritual practices to help them move from tension to calm. These tales demonstrate the significant influence that spiritual practices may have on mental health and show how every journey is different but related. In order to inspire readers to think about their own experiences and how they may apply these realizations to their lives, we will also provide a reflection section.

Narratives of Change

1. **Emma's Path to Mindfulness:**
   - Context: Emma was a busy business executive who frequently felt overburdened by stress at work. Her personal life and relationships were impacted by her anxiousness.

- o The Shift: Emma gained awareness of her thoughts and feelings by attending a mindfulness workshop and learning useful tools. She started implementing mindfulness exercises on a daily basis, like walking and attentive breathing.
- o Transformation: Emma observed a notable decrease in her anxiety levels over time. Being more present with her family and friends helped her make better decisions and enhance her relationships. Emma attributes the development of a balanced and satisfying existence to her journey towards mindfulness.

2. **James' Journey to Community Connection:**
   - o Background: James experienced feelings of loneliness and disconnection following his relocation to a new city for business. He yearned for a feeling of acceptance but had trouble locating a group that spoke to him.
   - o The Shift: James made the decision to enroll in a weekly meditation group in his community. He rapidly forged relationships with other members by practicing with them and discussing his experiences.
   - o Transformation: James felt more involved and supported as a result of his involvement. In addition to offering him emotional support, the friendships he made inspired him to continue practicing meditation. He discovered that a key component of spiritual development is interpersonal connection.

3. **Sofia's Experience with Nature:**
   - o Background: The stresses of everyday life frequently caused Sofia, an artist, to become creatively inhibited. Though she felt cut off from nature, she yearned for inspiration.
   - o The Shift: She made the spontaneous decision to go hiking in neighboring parks on the weekends. Disconnecting

from technology was difficult at first, but she quickly found serenity in the beauty of nature.

- o Transformation: Sofia's creativity was rekindled by her time spent outside. She started using aspects of the natural world in her artwork after nature became her muse. She was inspired to give workshops for others looking to connect with nature after the experience helped her manage stress.

4. Breathwork and Liam's Spiritual Awakening:
- o Background: Liam experienced a turbulent upbringing and carried unresolved pain into adulthood. He frequently experienced anxiety and emotional detachment.
- o The Shift: Liam learned about the transformational potential of his breath after participating in a breathwork session. He acquired methods for accessing and letting go of suppressed feelings.
- o Transformation: A vital component of Liam's recovery process was breathwork. He experienced emotional relief, clarity, and a stronger bond with his actual self. His life became more balanced and enjoyable as a result of this practice, which assisted him in addressing his prior traumas.

5. Nina's Acceptance of Gratitude:
- o Background: Nina had to deal with a number of difficult situations in her life, including the death of a loved one. She battled depression and hopelessness, frequently dwelling on her shortcomings.
- o The Shift: Nina started a daily gratitude notebook after being inspired by a friend. She changed her focus to the good things in her life by writing down three things for which she was thankful every evening.
- o Transformation: Nina observed a shift in her viewpoint throughout time. She developed resilience through the practice of gratitude, which allowed her to find joy even in

trying circumstances. She started talking about her experience and urging others to cultivate an attitude of thankfulness.

Reflection: Examining Your Own Path

Take some time to consider your own journey as you read these tales of transformation. To help you focus your thoughts, think about the following queries:

1. **What strikes a chord with you?**
   - o Think back on the tales that you found most moving. Which parts of their experiences inspire or resonate with you?

2. **What difficulties are you encountering?**
   - o List any emotional difficulties or tensions in your life. What effects have they had on your general wellbeing?

3. **Which behaviors appeal to you?**
   - o Consider the spiritual practices covered in this book. What kinds of practices appeal to you? How can they assist you in overcoming your obstacles?

4. **What are some ways to foster connection?**
   - o Think about your present network of support. Is it possible to strengthen your relationships with other people? In what ways could you interact with a spiritual community?

5. **What actions may you take to proceed?**
   - o Describe concrete actions you may take to make new routines a part of your everyday life. Building momentum can be facilitated by setting modest, attainable goals.

6. **For what do you feel thankful?**

- o Spend a moment appreciating the good things in your life. In the future, how can you develop a stronger sense of thankfulness?

7. How do you envision tranquility?
- o Imagine what you think serenity looks like. How does a happy, balanced existence feel? How would you like to achieve it?

In summary

This chapter's personal narratives demonstrate the various routes people have followed in search of spiritual fulfillment and emotional equilibrium. Although every path is different, they are all connected by resilience, community, and transformative practices.

As you reflect on your personal path, keep in mind that development is an ongoing process. Accept the actions you decide to take and give yourself permission to change. There are many chances for learning and connection along the nonlinear road from tension to calm. You are not traveling alone; a lot of people are walking with you, willing to share their knowledge and experiences while you look for your own way to happiness and contentment.

Conclusion

Let's take a moment to review the main ideas discussed throughout the book as we get to the end of our trip from tension to calm:

1. Understanding Stress and Its Impact: We looked at what stress is, how it affects our bodies and minds, and how long-term stress can impair our wellbeing.
2. The Relationship Between Spirituality and Emotional Health: Drawing on research showing the advantages of spiritual activities, we looked at how spirituality can improve emotional resilience.

3. Meditation, Prayer, and Mindfulness: While mindfulness exercises help us to interact with the present moment and lower stress, meditation and prayer provide avenues to inner peace.
4. Yoga and Breathwork: We explored yoga as a comprehensive method of bringing the body, mind, and spirit together as well as breathwork methods that use the power of our breath to control our emotions and lessen worry.
5. Gratitude and Affirmations: We talked about how these techniques can change our viewpoint and promote emotional equilibrium, highlighting the transformational potential of gratitude and positive affirmations.
6. Spiritual Rituals and Nature Connection: We discussed the significance of rituals in spiritual practice as well as the potent healing benefits of spending time in nature.
7. Creating a Supportive Community: We discussed how communities play a part in our spiritual development and provided advice on how to establish and maintain deep relationships.
8. Personal Transformation Stories: We demonstrated the significant influence that spiritual practices may have on people's lives with experiences from real life, highlighting the fact that everyone can undergo transformation.

I urge you to keep using the spiritual practices that you find most effective as you go forward. The secret to maintaining emotional health is consistency. Incorporate these techniques into your everyday routine gradually, starting small. Every action you take matters, whether it's practicing meditation for a short while, keeping a gratitude diary every day, or participating in a community.

Concluding Reflections on the Lifelong Path

Recall that the path from stress to calm is a lifetime of discovery and development rather than a final destination. It's a dynamic process that is impacted by our relationships, experiences, and internal changes. As you travel this path, practice self-compassion and patience, and welcome any changes that may arise.

You could discover that your definition of serenity changes as you develop these habits and understandings. It's not just the lack of worry; it's also a deep sense of joy, acceptance, and inner calm that can live with life's obstacles. Your path will be entirely your own, full of epiphanies, connections, and changes.

Appendix

Recommended Resources for Further Reading and Practice

1. **Books:**

   o   *The Miracle of Mindfulness* by Thich Nhat Hanh

   o   *The Untethered Soul* by Michael A. Singer

   o   *The Gifts of Imperfection* by Brené Brown

   o   *The Heart of the Buddha's Teaching* by Thich Nhat Hanh

2. **Podcasts:**

   o   "On Being" with Krista Tippett

   o   "The Mindfulness Meditation Podcast" from the Rubin Museum of Art o "The Happiness Lab" with Dr. Laurie Santos

3. **Online Courses:**

   o Mindfulness-Based Stress Reduction (MBSR) programs

   o Yoga Teacher Training or online yoga classes (e.g., Yoga with Adriene)

   o Breathwork workshops (e.g., Transformational Breath)

List of Spiritual Retreats and Workshops

1. **Kripalu Center for Yoga & Health (Massachusetts, USA)**

   o Offers various workshops and retreats focused on yoga, mindfulness, and personal growth.

2. **Esalen Institute (California, USA)**

   o A retreat center offering workshops in personal development, spirituality, and holistic health.

3. **Spirit Rock Meditation Center (California, USA)**

   o Provides silent retreats and workshops focused on mindfulness and insight meditation.

4. **The Omega Institute (New York, USA)**

   o Hosts workshops on various spiritual practices, including yoga, meditation, and personal transformation.

5. **Brahma Kumaris (Global)**

   o Offers retreats and workshops focused on meditation, inner peace, and spiritual knowledge.

Journaling Prompts for Self-Reflection and Growth

1. **Daily Gratitude:** List three things you are grateful for each day and reflect on how they impact your emotional well-being.

2. **Stress Triggers:** Write about situations that trigger your stress. What emotions do they evoke, and how can you respond differently?

3. **Mindfulness Moments:** Reflect on moments during your day when you practiced mindfulness. What did you notice? How did it feel?

4. **Spiritual Practices:** What spiritual techniques resonate most with you? How can you incorporate them into your daily routine?

5. **Community Connections:** Reflect on your current support system. Who uplifts you? How can you deepen these connections?

6. **Personal Growth:** Write about a recent challenge you faced. What did you learn about yourself through this experience?

7. **Vision for Serenity:** Envision what a serene life looks like for you. What steps can you take to move closer to that vision?

As you embark on your journey, may you find peace, connection, and joy in the practices that resonate with you. The path to serenity is yours to explore, and every step you take is a testament to your commitment to personal and spiritual growth.